50 Unmissable Paleo Diet Recipes

Tasty and Incredibly Healthy Recipes to Enjoy your Diet and Lose Weight

Carol Galindo

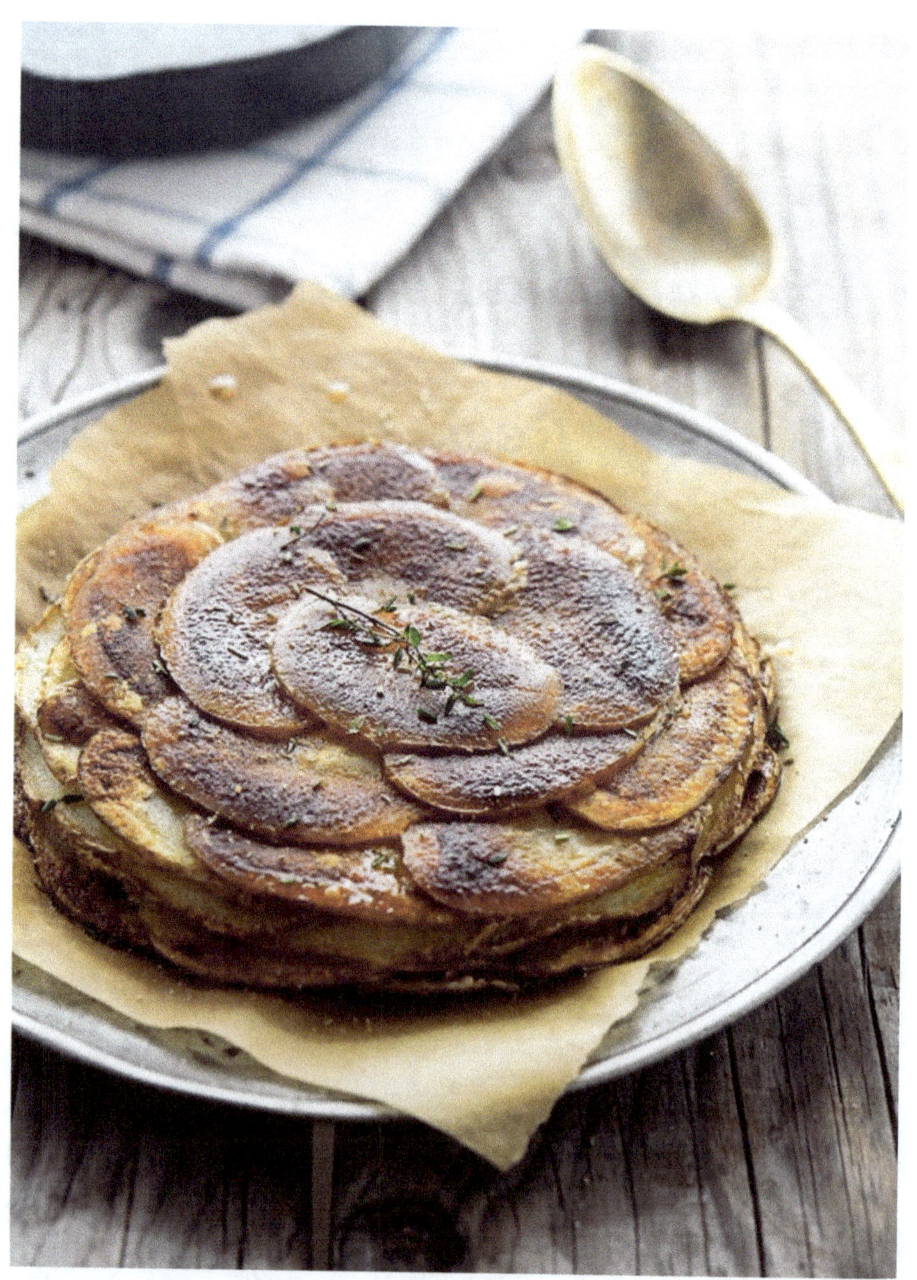

been executed to present accurate, up to date, and reliable, complete information. No warranties of any kind are declared or implied. Readers acknowledge that the author is not engaging in the rendering of legal, financial, medical or professional advice. The content within this book has been derived from various sources. Please consult a licensed professional before attempting any techniques outlined in this book.

By reading this document, the reader agrees that under no circumstances is the author responsible for any losses, direct or indirect, which are incurred as a result of the use of information contained within this document, including, but not limited to, — errors, omissions, or inaccuracies.

Table of Contents

Paleo Seafood and Fish Recipes

Dill Salmon

Preparation time: 10 minutes

Cooking time: 20 minutes

Servings: 4

Ingredients:

- 1 cup walnuts, chopped
- 4 salmon fillets, boneless
- ¼ cup lemon juice
- 2 tablespoons stevia
- 1 teaspoon dill, chopped
- A pinch of sea salt
- Black pepper to taste

- 1 tablespoon mustard

Directions:

1. In a bowl, mix the walnuts with mustard, stevia, lemon juice, a pinch of salt, black pepper and dill and stir well.

2. Spread this over salmon fillets, press well, place them on a lined baking sheet, place in the oven at 375 degrees F and bake for 20 minutes. Divide salmon between plates and serve with a side salad.

Nutritional value/serving: calories 446, fat 30,4, fiber 2,6, carbs 4,5, protein 42,9

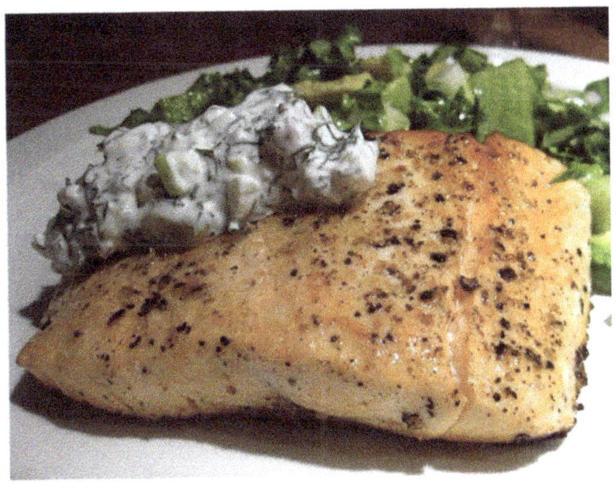

Calamari and Kale Mix

Preparation time: 15 minutes

Cooking time: 50 minutes

Servings: 4

Ingredients:

- 4 big calamari, tentacles separated and chopped
- 2 tablespoons parsley, chopped
- 5 ounces kale, chopped
- 2 garlic cloves, minced
- 1 red bell pepper, chopped
- 1 teaspoon oregano, dried
- 15 ounces homemade tomato puree
- Olive oil
- 1 yellow onion, chopped
- A pinch of sea salt
- Black pepper to taste

Directions:

1. Heat up a pan with some olive oil over medium heat, add onion and garlic, stir and cook for 2 minutes.

2. Add bell pepper, stir and cook for 3 minutes.

3. Add calamari tentacles, stir and cook for 6 minutes more.

4. Add kale, a pinch of sea salt and black pepper, stir, cook for a couple more minutes and take off heat.

5. Stuff calamari tubes with this mix and secure with toothpicks.

6. Heat up a pan with some olive oil over medium-high heat, add calamari, brown them for 2 minutes on each side and then mix with tomato puree.

7. Also add parsley, oregano and some black pepper to the pan, stir gently, cover, reduce heat to medium-low and simmer for 40 minutes.

8. Divide stuffed calamari on plates and serve.

Nutritional value/serving: calories 637, fat 23,7, fiber 6,3, carbs 57,9, protein 42,9

Maple Salmon

Preparation time: 10 minutes

Cooking time: 12 minutes

Servings: 4

Ingredients:

- 2 tablespoons dill, chopped
- 4 salmon fillets, boneless
- 2 tablespoons chives, chopped
- 1/3 cup maple syrup
- A drizzle of olive oil
- 3 tablespoons balsamic vinegar
- A pinch of sea salt
- Black pepper to taste
- Lime wedges for serving

Directions:

1. Heat up a pan with the oil over medium-high heat, add fish fillets, season them with a pinch of sea salt

and black pepper, cook for 3 minutes, cover pan and
cook for 6 minutes more.

2. Add balsamic vinegar and maple syrup and cook for 3
   minutes basting fish with this mix.

3. Add dill and chives, cook for 1 minute, divide the fish
   between plates and serve with lime wedges on the
   side.

Nutritional value/serving: calories 346, fat 14,7, fiber 0,7,
carbs 20,4, protein 35

Mustard Cod

Preparation time: 10 minutes

Cooking time: 20 minutes

Servings: 4

Ingredients:

- 1 tablespoon cilantro, chopped
- 4 medium cod fillets, boneless
- ¼ cup ghee
- 2 garlic cloves, minced
- 2 tablespoons olive oil
- 2 tablespoons lemon juice
- 3 tablespoons prosciutto, chopped
- 1 teaspoon Dijon mustard
- 1 shallot, chopped
- A pinch of sea salt
- Black pepper to taste

Directions:

1. In a bowl, mix mustard with ghee, garlic, cilantro, shallot, lemon juice, prosciutto, salt and pepper and whisk well.

2. Heat up a pan with the oil over medium-high heat, add the fish fillets, season them with some black pepper and cook for 4 minutes on each side.

3. Spread mustard and ghee mix over fish, transfer everything to a lined baking sheet, place in the oven at 425 degrees F and bake for 10 minutes.

4. Divide fish between plates and serve.

Nutritional value/serving: calories 279, fat 21,2, fiber 0,1, carbs 1,3, protein 21,7

Halibut and Peppers Slaw

Preparation time: 15 minutes

Cooking time: 10 minutes

Servings: 4

Ingredients:

- 4 medium halibut fillets, skinless, boneless

- 2 teaspoons olive oil

- 4 teaspoons lemon juice

- 1 garlic clove, minced

- 1 teaspoon sweet paprika

- A pinch of sea salt

- Black pepper to taste

For the salsa:

- ¼ cup green onions, chopped

- 1 cup red bell pepper, chopped

- 4 teaspoons oregano, chopped

- 1 small habanero pepper, chopped

- 1 garlic clove, minced

- ¼ cup lemon juice

Directions:

1. In a bowl, mix red bell pepper with habanero, green onion, ¼ cup lemon juice, 1 garlic clove, oregano, a pinch of sea salt and black pepper, stir well and keep in the fridge for now.

2. In a large bowl, mix paprika, olive oil, 1 garlic clove and 4 teaspoons lemon juice and stir well.

3. Add fish, rub well, cover bowl and leave aside for 10 minutes.

4. Place marinated fish under preheated broiler over medium-high heat, season with a pinch of sea salt and black pepper, cook for 4 minutes on each side and divide between plates.

5. Top fish with the salsa you've made earlier and serve.

Nutritional value/serving: calories 402, fat 8,7, fiber 0,2, carbs 0,6, protein 75,7

Salmon Rolls

Preparation time: 10 minutes

Cooking time: 20 minutes

Servings: 4

Ingredients:

- 6 cabbage leaves, sliced in half
- 4 medium salmon steaks, skinless
- 2 red bell peppers, chopped
- Some coconut oil
- 1 yellow onion, chopped
- A pinch of sea salt
- Black pepper to taste

Directions:

1. Put water in a large saucepan, bring to a boil over medium-high heat, add cabbage leaves, blanch them

for 2 minutes, transfer to a bowl filled with cold water and pat dry.

2. Season salmon steaks with a pinch of sea salt and black pepper to taste and wrap each in 3 cabbage leaf halves.

3. Heat up a pan with some coconut oil over medium-high heat, add onion and bell pepper, stir and cook for 4 minutes.

4. Add wrapped salmon, place pan in the oven at 350 degrees F and bake for 12 minutes.

5. Divide salmon and veggies between plates and serve.

Nutritional value/serving: calories 271, fat 11,2, fiber 2, carbs 8,4, protein 35,7

Paleo Vegetables Recipes

Salmon Stuffed Peppers

Preparation time: 10 minutes

Cooking time: 10 minutes

Servings: 4

Ingredients:

- 2 bell peppers, tops cut off, cut in halves and seeds removed
- 1 tablespoon capers, chopped
- 2 tablespoons tomato puree
- 4 ounces cooked salmon
- 1 scallion, chopped
- 1 tomato, chopped
- Black pepper to taste

Directions:

1. Place bell pepper halves on a lined baking sheet, place under a preheated broiler on medium-high heat, broil for 4 minutes and then leave them aside to cool down.

2. Meanwhile, in a bowl mix capers with tomato puree, salmon, tomato, black pepper and scallion and stir well.

3. Stuff bell peppers with this mix, place under preheated broiler again and cook for 5 minutes.

4. Divide between plates and serve.

Nutritional value/serving: calories 64, fat 2, fiber 1,3, carbs 6,2, protein 6,5

Garlic and Liver Stuffed Peppers

Preparation time: 10 minutes

Cooking time: 15 minutes

Servings: 4

Ingredients:

- 3 small shallots, peeled, chopped

- 1 white onion, chopped

- ½ pound chicken livers, chopped

- 4 garlic cloves, chopped

- 4 bell peppers, tops cut off and seeds removed

- A pinch of sea salt

- Black pepper to taste

- ½ teaspoon lemon zest, grated

- ¼ teaspoon thyme, chopped

- ¼ teaspoon dill, chopped

- A drizzle of olive oil

- A handful parsley, chopped

Directions:

1. Heat up a pan over medium heat, add chopped shallots, stir for 5 minutes.

2. Add onion and garlic, stir and cook for 2 minutes.

3. Add livers, a pinch of salt and black pepper, stir, cook for 5 minutes and take off heat.

4. Transfer this to a food processor, blend well, transfer to a bowl and aside for 10 minutes.

5. Add thyme, oil, parsley, lemon zest and dill, stir well and stuff each bell pepper with this mix.

6. Serve right away.

Nutritional value/serving: calories 188, fat 7,6, fiber 2,5, carbs 15,6, protein 16,1

Almond Eggplant Bake

Preparation time: 10 minutes

Cooking time: 30 minutes

Servings: 3

Ingredients:

- 2 eggplants, sliced
- A pinch of sea salt
- Black pepper to taste
- 1 cup almonds, ground
- 1 teaspoon garlic, minced
- 2 teaspoons olive oil

Directions:

1. Grease a baking dish with some of the oil and arrange eggplant slices on it.
2. Season them with a pinch of salt and some black pepper and leave them aside for 10 minutes.

3. In a food processor, mix almonds with the rest of the oil, garlic, a pinch of salt and black pepper and blend well.

4. Spread this over eggplant slices, place in the oven at 425 degrees F and bake for 30 minutes.

5. Divide between plates and serve.

Nutritional value/serving: calories 303, fat 19,6, fiber 16,9, carbs 28,6, protein 10,3

Maple Eggplant Rounds

Preparation time: 10 minutes

Cooking time: 40 minutes

Servings: 3

Ingredients:

- 5 medium eggplants, sliced into rounds
- 1 teaspoon thyme, chopped
- 2 tablespoons balsamic vinegar
- 1 teaspoon mustard
- 2 garlic cloves, minced
- ½ cup olive oil
- Black pepper to taste
- A pinch of sea salt
- 1 teaspoon maple syrup

Directions:

1. In a bowl, mix vinegar with thyme, mustard, garlic, oil, salt, pepper and maple syrup and whisk very well.

2. Arrange eggplant round on a lined baking sheet, place in the oven at 425 degrees F and roast for 40 minutes.

3. Divide eggplants between plates and serve.

Nutritional value/serving: calories 533, fat 35,6, fiber 32,6, carbs 56,5, protein 9,4

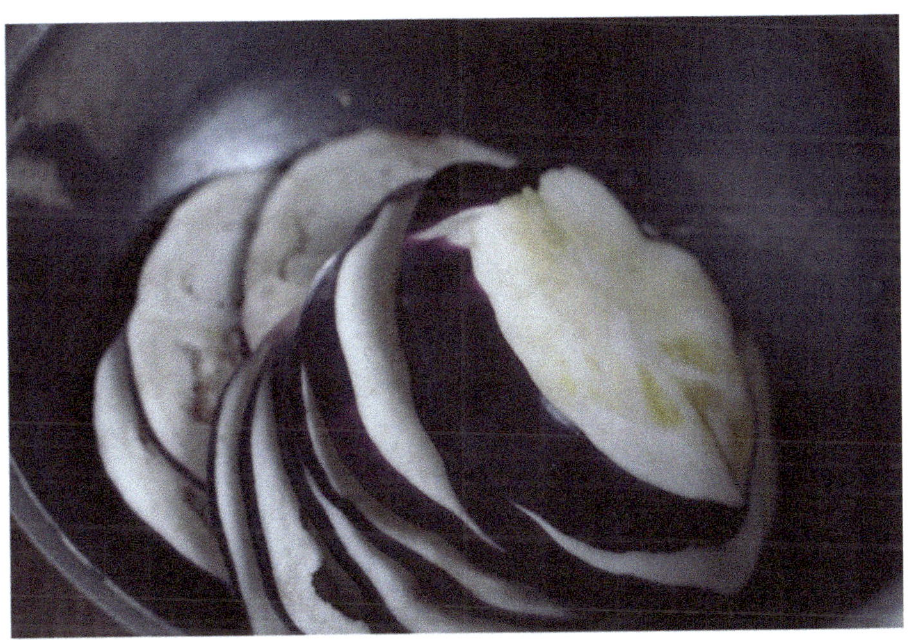

Eggplant and Beef Bake

Preparation time: 10 minutes

Cooking time: 50 minutes

Servings: 4

Ingredients:

- 2 eggplants, sliced

- 3 tablespoons olive oil

- 1 pound beef, ground

- 1 garlic clove, minced

- ¾ cup tomato sauce

- ½ bunch basil, chopped

- A pinch of sea salt

- Black pepper to taste

Directions:

1. Heat up a pan with 1 tablespoon oil over medium-high heat, add eggplant slices, cook for 5 minutes on

each side, transfer them to paper towels, drain grease and leave them aside.

2. Heat up another pan with the rest of the oil over medium-high heat, add garlic, stir and cook for 1 minute.

3. Add beef, stir and cook for 5 minutes more.

4. Add tomato sauce, stir and cook for 5 minutes more.

5. Add a pinch of sea salt and black pepper, stir, take off heat and mix with basil.

6. Place one layer of eggplant slices into a baking dish, add one layer of beef mix and repeat with the rest of the eggplant slices and beef.

7. Place in the oven at 350 degrees F and bake for 30 minutes.

8. Leave eggplant casserole to cool down, slice and serve.

Nutritional value/serving: calories 382, fat 18,2, fiber 10,4, carbs 18,9, protein 37,8

Eggplant and Green Onion Sauce

Preparation time: 10 minutes

Cooking time: 10 minutes

Servings: 4

Ingredients:

- 2 tablespoons avocado oil

- 2 garlic cloves, minced

- 3 eggplants, cut into halves and thinly sliced

- 1 red chili pepper, chopped

- 1 green onion stalk, chopped

- 1 tablespoon ginger, grated

- 1 tablespoon coconut aminos

- 1 tablespoon balsamic vinegar

Directions:

1. Heat up a pan with half of the oil over medium-high heat, add eggplant slices, cook for 2 minutes, flip, cook for 3 minutes more and transfer to a plate.

2. Heat up the pan with the rest of the oil over medium heat, add chili pepper, garlic, green onions and ginger, stir and cook for 1 minute. Return eggplant slices to the pan, stir and cook for 1 minute.

3. Add coconut aminos and vinegar, stir, divide between plates and serve.

Nutritional value/serving: calories 123, fat 1,7, fiber 15,2, carbs 26,7, protein 4,4

Paleo Salad Recipes

Chicken and Nuts Salad

Preparation time: 10 minutes

Cooking time: 0 minutes

Servings: 2

Ingredients:

- 1 and ½ tablespoons vinegar

- 3 tablespoons olive oil

- 1 teaspoon thyme, dried

- 2 tablespoons macadamia nuts, chopped

- A pinch of sea salt

- Black pepper to taste

- ¾ cup chicken, cooked and shredded

- 3 tablespoons onion, chopped

- ¼ cup carrot, grated

- 4 radishes, chopped

- ½ cup red cabbage, shredded

- ½ cup green cabbage, shredded

Directions:

1. In a salad bowl, mix chicken with macadamia nuts, carrot, onion, radishes, green and red cabbage.

2. In a bowl, mix vinegar with oil, a pinch of salt, black pepper and thyme and whisk well.

3. Add this to salad, toss to coat and serve.

Nutritional value/serving: calories 398, fat 29,3, fiber 2,2, carbs 5,7, protein 16,5

Broccoli and Mushroom Salad

Preparation time: 10 minutes

Cooking time: 0 minutes

Servings: 2

Ingredients:

- 3 carrots, sliced

- 1 cup broccoli, chopped

- 1/3 cup mushrooms, sliced

- 2 tablespoons walnuts, chopped

- 3 tablespoons red onion, chopped

- 3 tablespoons black olives, pitted and chopped

- A pinch of sea salt

- Black pepper to taste

- 1 teaspoon mustard

- 3 tablespoons olive oil

- 1 and ½ tablespoons balsamic vinegar

Directions:

1. In a salad bowl, mix carrots with olives, onion, walnuts, mushrooms and broccoli.

2. In a small bowl, mix oil with vinegar, mustard, salt and pepper and whisk well.

3. Add this to salad, toss to coat and serve.

Nutritional value/serving: calories 315, fat 27,6, fiber 5, carbs 16, protein 5

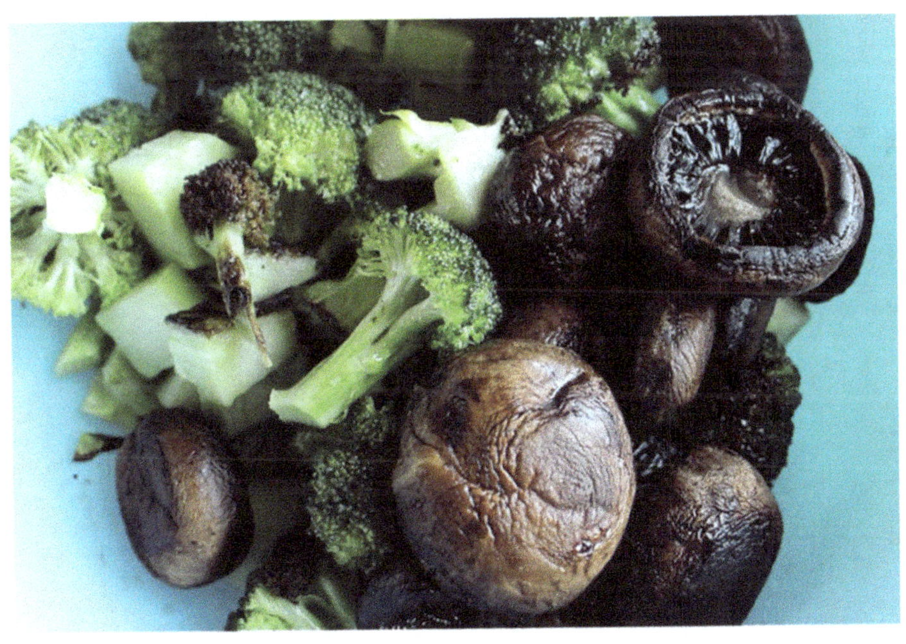

Salmon and Strawberries Salad

Preparation time: 10 minutes

Cooking time: 8 minutes

Servings: 4

Ingredients:

- 1 pound salmon fillet
- 2 tablespoons olive oil
- ¼ teaspoon coriander, ground
- ½ teaspoon cumin, ground
- 1 teaspoon chili powder
- ¼ teaspoon paprika
- A pinch of sea salt
- Black pepper to taste
- 6 strawberries, chopped
- ¼ cup red onion, chopped
- 1 jalapeno, chopped
- Juice from 1 lime

- 1 garlic clove, minced

- 5 ounces baby arugula

- ½ avocado, pitted, peeled and chopped

- 3 radishes, chopped

For the vinaigrette:

- ¼ cup balsamic vinegar

- 1/3 cup olive oil

- ½ teaspoon lemon zest

- 3 strawberries, chopped

- 1 tablespoon lemon juice

- 1 and ½ tablespoons maple syrup

- 1 and ½ tablespoons mustard

Directions:

1. In a bowl, mix 2 tablespoons oil with coriander, cumin, chili powder, paprika, a pinch of salt and black pepper to taste and whisk well.

2. Brush salmon with this mix, place under preheated pan over medium-high heat, cook for 6 minutes skin

side down, flip, cook for 2 minutes more, transfer to a cutting board, leave aside to cool down, cut into medium pieces and transfer to a bowl.

3. Add radishes, avocado, 6 strawberries, garlic, arugula, red onion, jalapeno and lime juice and toss gently.

4. In another bowl, mix 1/3 cup oil with 3 strawberries, vinegar, lemon zest, 1 tablespoon lemon juice, maple syrup and mustard and whisk very well.

5. Add this to salad, toss to coat and serve.

Nutritional value/serving: calories 458, fat 37,7, fiber 3,3, carbs 10,4, protein 23,9

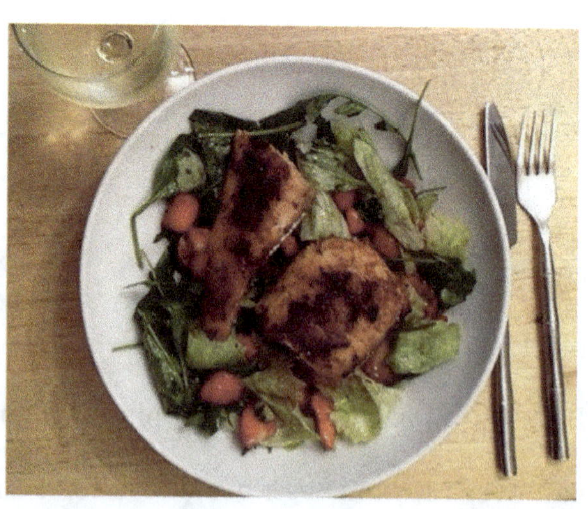

Coconut Potato Salad

Preparation time: 10 minutes

Cooking time: 4 minutes

Servings: 4

Ingredients:

For the salad dressing:

- 1 tablespoon parsley, chopped

- 1/3 cup cashew butter

- 1 tablespoon sesame seeds

- ½ cup green onion, chopped

- 2 tablespoons tamari sauce

- 2 tablespoons lemon juice

- 2 tablespoons vinegar

- A pinch of sea salt

- Black pepper to taste

- 2 garlic cloves, minced

- 1/3 cup coconut milk

- ¼ cup avocado oil

For the salad:

- 2 tablespoons water

- 3 sweet potatoes, cut with a spiralizer

- 1 tablespoon parsley, chopped

Directions:

1. In a blender, mix cashew butter with 1 tablespoon parsley, green onion, sesame seeds, vinegar, tamari sauce, lemon juice, garlic, coconut milk, a pinch of salt and black pepper and pulse well. Add the oil gradually and blend again well.

2. Put sweet potato noodles in a bowl, add the water, place in your microwave and steam at High for 4 minutes.

3. Drain potato noodles, transfer to a bowl and add 1 tablespoon parsley.

4. Add dressing, toss to coat and serve.

Nutritional value/serving: calories 296, fat 13,9, fiber 6,7, carbs 39,3, protein 6,2

Beet and Walnuts Salad

Preparation time: 10 minutes

Cooking time: 0 minutes

Servings: 2

Ingredients:

- 2 beetroots, cooked, peeled and cut into medium pieces
- 1/3 cup walnuts, chopped
- ¼ teaspoon cinnamon powder
- ½ teaspoon maple syrup
- 2 tablespoons olive oil
- 1 tablespoon vinegar
- ½ teaspoon mustard
- 3 cups salad leaves, torn
- A pinch of sea salt
- Black pepper to taste

Directions:

1. In a salad bowl, combine all the ingredients, toss and serve.

Nutritional value/serving: calories 336, fat 26,9, fiber 3,5, carbs 20,2, protein 9,5

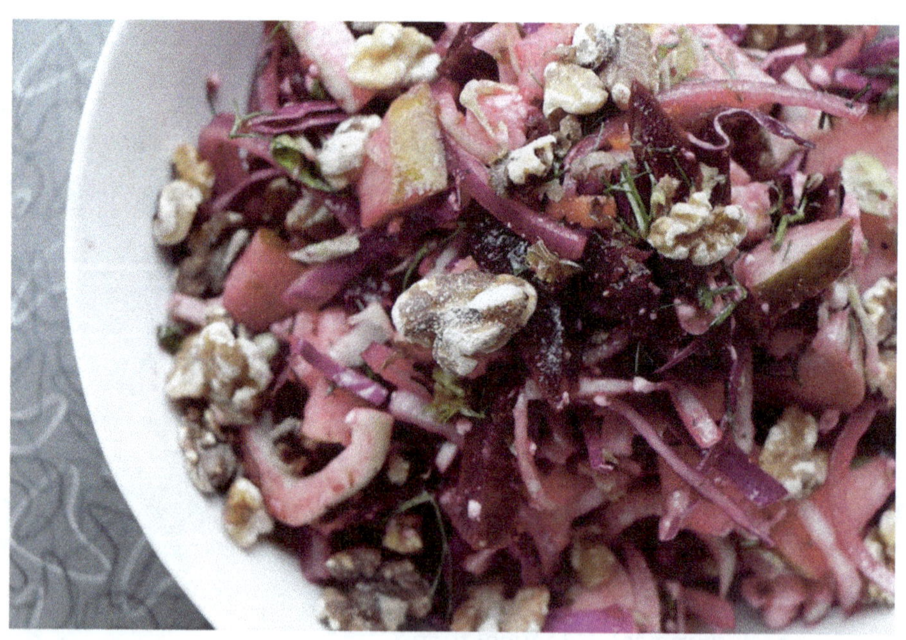

Turkey and Arugula Salad

Preparation time: 10 minutes

Cooking time: 20 minutes

Servings: 4

Ingredients:

- 4 cups arugula

- 1 tablespoon rosemary, chopped

- 2 green onions, chopped

- 10 ounce turkey meat, sliced

- 1 tablespoon olive oil

- 2 garlic cloves, minced

- 4 sweet potatoes, peeled and cubed

- A pinch of sea salt

- Black pepper to taste

For the salad dressing:

- 2 teaspoons mustard

- 2 tablespoons apple vinegar

- 4 tablespoons olive oil

- ½ teaspoon lemon juice

Directions:

1. Heat up a pan with the olive oil over medium heat, add sweet potatoes, stir and cook for 7 minutes.

2. Add a pinch of salt, black pepper, rosemary and garlic, stir and cook for 6 minutes more.

3. Add turkey meat slices, stir, cook for 3 minutes, take off heat, cool down and transfer everything to a salad bowl.

4. Add green onions and arugula and stir.

5. In a small bowl, mix olive oil with lemon juice, vinegar, mustard and some black pepper and whisk well.

6. Add this to salad, toss to coat and serve.

Nutritional value/serving: calories 468, fat 22,1, fiber 7,3, carbs 44,7, protein 24,3

Paleo Dessert Recipes

Grapefruit Cream

Preparation time: 10 minutes

Cooking time: 0 minutes

Servings: 2

Ingredients:

- 1 pounds grapefruit jelly

- ½ pound coconut cream

- A handful fresh berries for serving

- A handful nuts, roughly chopped for serving

Directions:

1. In a food processor, combine grapefruit jelly with coconut cream and blend well.

2. Add berries and nuts, toss gently, transfer to dessert
cups and serve right away!

Nutritional value/serving: calories 558, fat 36,6, carbs 55,3,
fiber 4,6, protein 7,8

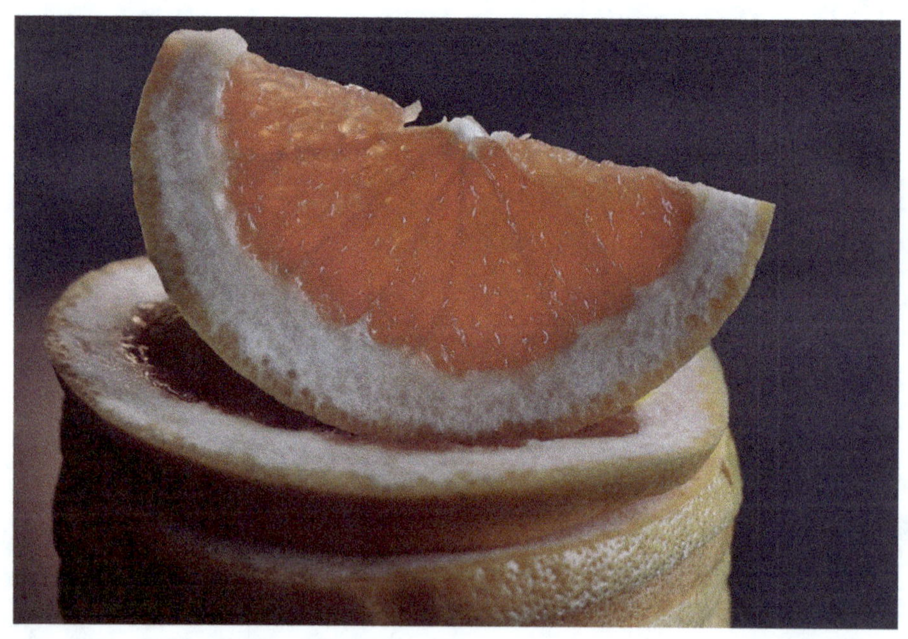

Figs and Sauce

Preparation time: 10 minutes

Cooking time: 5 minutes

Servings: 4

Ingredients:

- 2 tablespoons coconut butter
- 12 figs cut in halves
- ¼ cup maple syrup
- 1 cup almonds, toasted and chopped

Directions:

1. Heat up a saucepan with the butter over medium-high heat and stir until it melts.
2. Add maple syrup and figs, stir well and cook for about 5 minutes.
3. Add almonds, stir gently and take off heat.
4. Transfer to dessert bowls and serve right away!

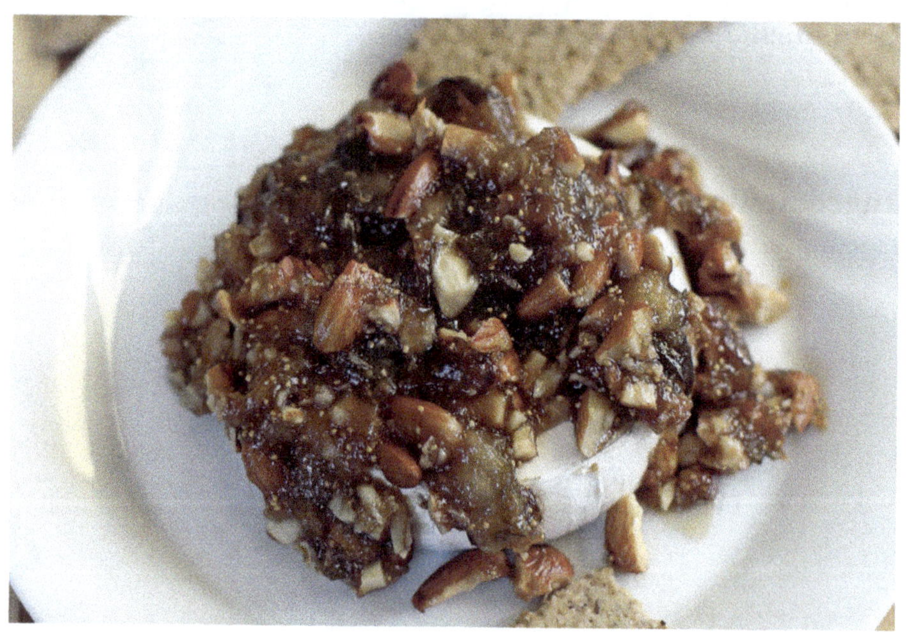

Maple Cake

Preparation time: 10 minutes

Cooking time: 30 minutes

Servings: 4

Ingredients:

- 1 and ½ cups coconut flour
- 1 teaspoon cinnamon
- 1,5 teaspoon baking soda
- ¾ cup maple syrup
- 1 cup tomatoes chopped
- ½ cup extra virgin olive oil
- 2 tablespoon apple cider vinegar

Directions:

1. In a bowl, mix flour with baking soda, cinnamon and maple syrup and stir well.

2. In another bowl, mix tomatoes with olive oil and vinegar and stir well.

3. Combine the 2 mixtures, stir well and pour everything into a greased round pan.

4. Place cake in the oven at 375 degrees F and bake for 30 minutes.

5. Take cake out of the oven, leave aside to cool down, transfer to a platter, cut and serve it.

Nutritional value: calories 609, fat 31,1, carbs 80,1, fiber 23,6, protein 8,1

Spinach and Apple Smoothie

Preparation time: 10 minutes

Cooking time: 0 minutes

Servings: 3

Ingredients:

- 1 big green apple, cored and cut into medium cubes
- 1 cup baby spinach
- 1 tablespoon pure maple syrup
- A pinch of cardamom
- ½ teaspoon cinnamon
- ½ teaspoon vanilla extract

Directions:

1. Put apple cubes in a food processor.
2. Add spinach, maple syrup, vanilla extract, cardamom and cinnamon and blend until you obtain a smooth cream.

3. Pour into 2 glasses and serve right away!

Nutritional value/serving: calories 62, fat 0,2, fiber 2,2, carbs 15,6, protein 0,5

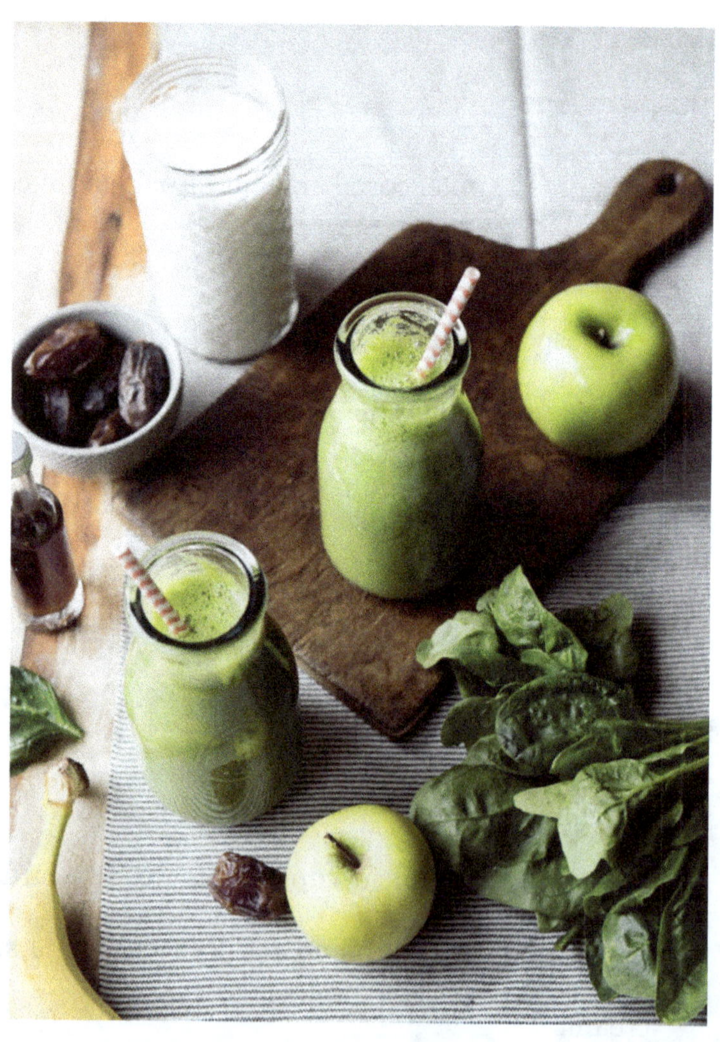

Paleo Snacks and Appetizer Recipes

Turkey Stuffed Mushrooms

Preparation time: 10 minutes

Cooking time: 30 minutes

Servings: 4

Ingredients:

- 1 pound turkey meat, chopped
- 1 pound big white mushroom caps, stems separated and chopped
- 3 tablespoons coconut oil
- 1 yellow onion, chopped
- A pinch of black pepper

Directions:

1. Heat up a pan with 2 tablespoons oil over medium heat, add mushrooms stems, stir and cook them for 3 minutes.
2. Add the rest of the oil, onion and a pinch of black pepper, stir and cook for 7 minutes.
3. Transfer this mix to a bowl, add turkey meat and stir well.
4. Stuff mushrooms with this mix, place them on a lined baking sheet and bake in the oven at 400 degrees F for 30 minutes.
5. Arrange mushrooms on a platter and serve them.

Nutritional value/serving: calories 317, fat 15,9, fiber 1,9, carbs 6,3, protein 37,2

Turmeric Mushroom Skewers

Preparation time: 20 minutes

Cooking time: 10 minutes

Servings: 4

Ingredients:

- 10 mushroom caps

- ½ teaspoon chili powder

- 1 cup broccoli florets

- 1 teaspoon garam masala

- 1 teaspoon ginger and garlic paste

- ½ teaspoon turmeric powder

- A drizzle of olive oil

- A pinch of sea salt

- Black pepper to taste

Directions:

1. In a bowl, mix chili powder, garam masala, ginger paste, turmeric, salt, pepper and oil and stir.

2. Add mushroom caps and broccoli florets, toss to coat well and keep in the fridge for 20 minutes.

3. Arrange these on skewers, place them on preheated grill over medium-high heat, cook for 5 minutes on each side and transfer to a platter.

4. Serve them as an appetizer.

Nutritional value/serving: calories 20, fat 1,5, fiber 0,5, carbs 1,3, protein 0,9

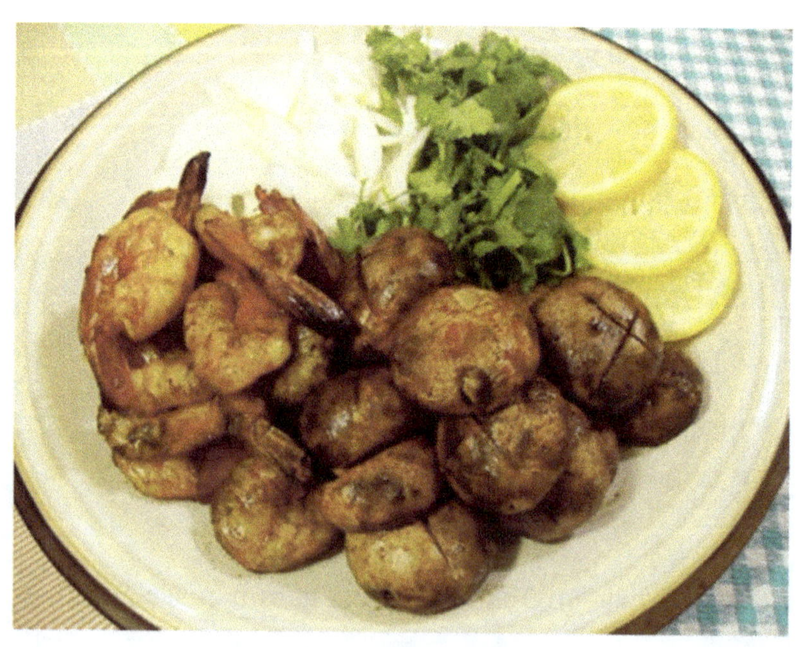

Zucchini Wraps

Preparation time: 10 minutes

Cooking time: 5 minutes

Servings: 4

Ingredients:

- 3 zucchinis, thinly sliced lengthwise
- 10 ounces turkey meat, cooked, sliced into thin strips
- ½ cup sun-dried tomatoes, drained and chopped
- 4 tablespoons raspberry vinegar
- ½ cup basil, chopped
- A pinch of sea salt
- Black pepper to taste

Directions:

1. Place zucchini slices in a bowl, sprinkle a pinch of sea salt and vinegar over them and leave aside for 10 minutes.

2. Drain well and season with black pepper to taste.

3. Divide turkey slices, chopped sun dried tomatoes and basil over zucchini ones, roll each and secure with a toothpick and arrange them on a lined baking sheet.

4. Place in the oven at 400 degrees F for 5 minutes, then arrange them on a platter and serve as an appetizer.

Nutritional value/serving: calories 152, fat 3,9, fiber 1,9, carbs 6, protein 22,8

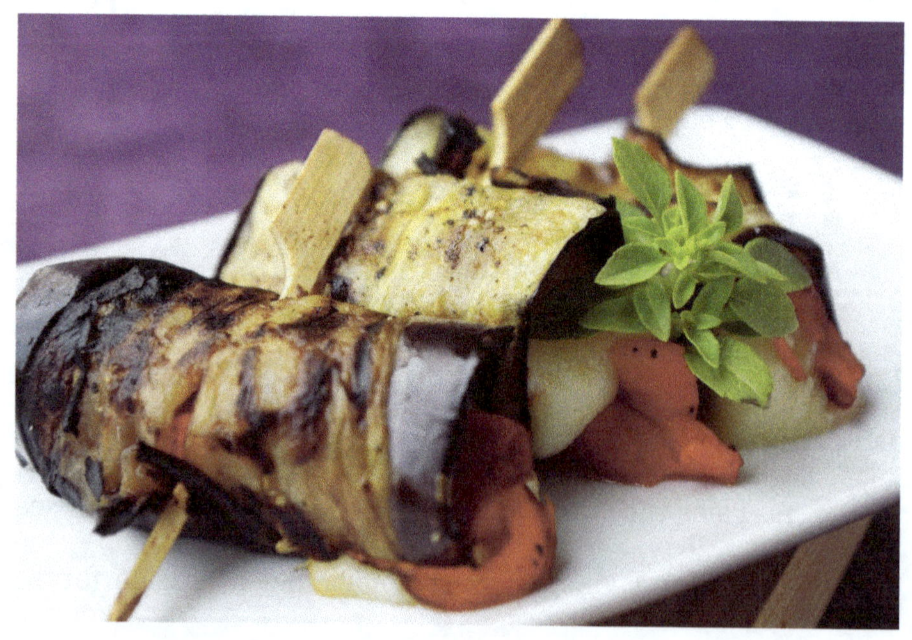

Turkey Bites

Preparation time: 10 minutes

Cooking time: 25 minutes

Servings: 6

Ingredients:

- 20 ounces ground turkey
- 2 eggs, whisked
- 1 cup cauliflower, riced
- 1 and ½ tablespoon coconut oil
- ½ teaspoon baking soda
- 1 teaspoon apple cider vinegar
- ¼ cup coconut flour
- 1 teaspoon red pepper sauce
- A pinch of sea salt
- ¼ teaspoon smoked paprika
- ½ teaspoon mustard powder
- A pinch of chili powder

- 2 teaspoons jalapenos, chopped

Directions:

1. In a bowl, mix the cauliflower rice with the coconut flour, eggs, oil, red pepper sauce, mustard, salt, chili powder, paprika and jalapenos and stir.

2. Add the baking soda and the vinegar and stir well again.

3. Place 12 spoonfuls of this mix on a lined baking sheet, put 1 tsp of turkey mince on each cauliflower circle, and top with other 12 spoonfuls of cauliflower mix.

4. Seal edges, place in the oven at 400 degrees F and bake for 30 minutes.

5. Arrange on a platter and serve them.

Nutritional value/serving: calories 240, fat 15, fiber 0,8, carbs 1,6, protein 28,2

Paleo Recipes for Breakfast

Potato Cups

Preparation time: 10 minutes

Cooking time: 30 minutes

Servings: 2

Ingredients:

- 3 small shallots

- 4 eggs

- ½ yellow onion, chopped

- 1 sweet potato, peeled and chopped

- 1 tablespoon olive oil

- A pinch of sea salt and black pepper

Directions:

1. Heat up a pan over medium-high heat, add the shallots, cook for 5 minutes, drain excess oil on paper

towels and fill 4 muffin molds with it.

2. Crack an egg into each shallot cup, season with salt
    and pepper, place in the oven at 375 degrees F and
    bake for 15 minutes.

3. Heat up a pan with the oil over medium-high heat,
    add the onion and sweet potato, stir and cook for 4
    minutes.

4. Divide egg cups between plates and serve with the
    sweet potato mix on the side.

Nutritional value/serving: calories 266, fat 15,9, fiber 2,5,
carbs 19,3, protein 13,2

Coconut Muffins

Preparation time: 10 minutes

Cooking time: 25 minutes

Servings: 10

Ingredients:

- ½ teaspoon baking soda

- 2 and ½ cups almond flour

- 1 tablespoon vanilla extract

- ¼ cup coconut oil, melted

- ¼ cup coconut milk

- 2 eggs, whisked

- 3 tablespoons cinnamon powder

- 1 cup blackberries

Directions:

1. In a bowl, mix all the ingredients and combine them well.

2. Divide this into lined muffin cups, bake at 350 degrees F for 25 minutes, divide between plates and serve them for breakfast.

Nutritional value/serving: calories 154, fat 7,8, fiber 0,9, carbs 7,2, protein 2,5

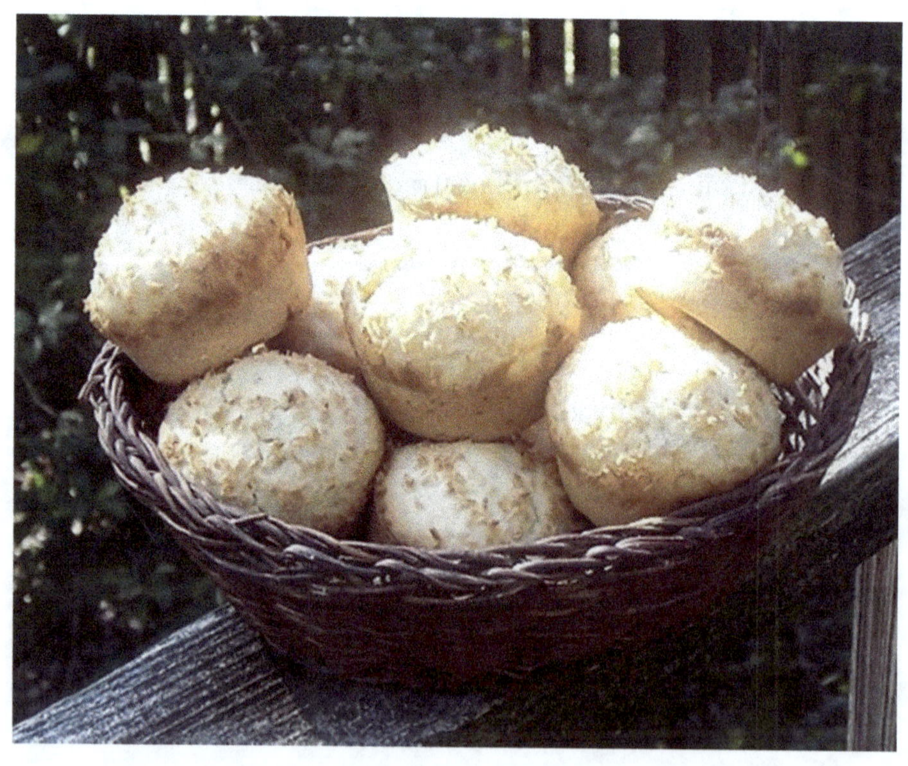

Ginger Berry Muffins

Preparation time: 10 minutes

Cooking time: 25 minutes

Servings: 10

Ingredients:

- 1 and ¼ cup almond meal

- 3 tablespoons flax meal

- ¾ cup coconut flour

- 1 teaspoon baking soda

- 2 teaspoons pumpkin pie spice

- ½ teaspoon nutmeg, ground

- ½ teaspoon ginger powder

- 5 eggs, whisked

- ¼ cup coconut oil, melted

- ¼ cup coconut sugar

- 1 cup pumpkin puree

- 1 cup blueberries

Directions:

1. In a bowl, mix all the ingredients and combine them well.

2. Divide this into a lined muffin tray, place in the oven at 350 degrees F and bake for 25 minutes.

3. Leave your muffins to cool down, divide them between plates and serve.

Nutritional value/serving: calories 179, fat 10,2, fiber 6,1, carbs 18,8, protein 5,3

Cocoa and Coconut Muffins

Preparation time: 10 minutes

Cooking time: 30 minutes

Servings: 8

Ingredients:

- 4 eggs
- ¼ cup coconut sugar
- ¼ cup melted ghee
- ¼ cup coconut milk
- 1 cup coconut flour
- 1 teaspoon baking soda
- ¼ cup cocoa powder
- 1 zucchini, grated
- 3 ounces cocoa powder
- 1 ounce cocoa butter
- 1 teaspoon vanilla extract

Directions:

1. In a bowl, combine all the ingredients and stir well.

2. Divide into a lined muffin tray and bake in the oven at 350 degrees F for 30 minutes.

3. Serve your muffins for breakfast.

Nutritional value/serving: calories 243, fat 11,6, fiber 11,6, carbs 26,7, protein 7,5

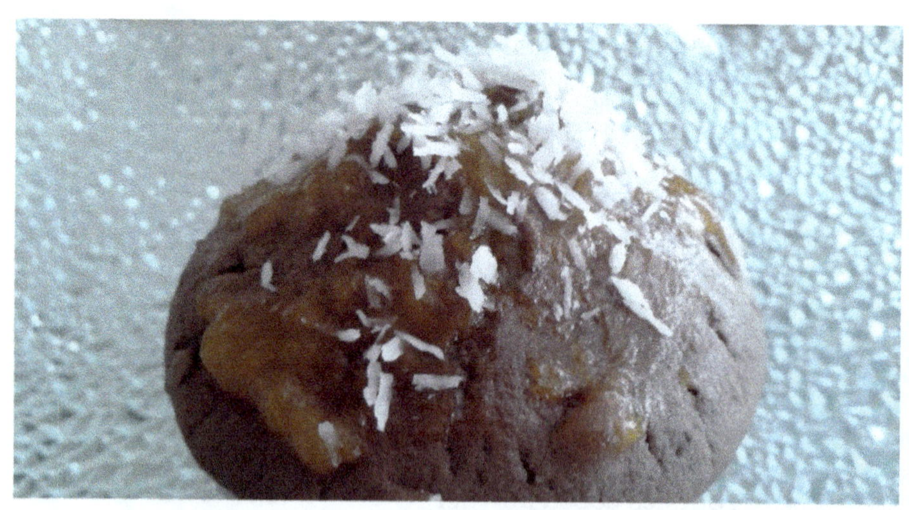

Shallot and Coconut Muffins

Preparation time: 10 minutes

Cooking time: 25 minutes

Servings: 12

Ingredients:

- 6 small shallots, peeled, chopped
- 1 yellow onion, chopped
- 4 avocados, pitted, peeled and mashed
- 4 eggs
- ½ cup coconut flour
- 1 cup coconut milk
- ½ teaspoon baking soda
- A pinch of sea salt and black pepper

Directions:

1. Heat up a pan over medium-high heat, add the shallots and onion, stir and cook for 5 minutes.

2. In a bowl, mix the avocados with the eggs, salt, black pepper, milk, baking soda and coconut flour and stir.

3. Add the shallots and onions, stir well again and divide into muffin pans.

4. Place in the oven at 350 degrees F and bake for 20 minutes.

5. Divide the muffins between plates and serve.

Nutritional value/serving: calories 252, fat 20,3, fiber 9,1, carbs 15,6, protein 5,2

Pepper and Spinach Eggs Mix

Preparation time: 10 minutes

Cooking time: 15 minutes

Servings: 4

Ingredients:

- 2 eggs, whisked
- 1 tablespoon ghee, melted
- A pinch of black pepper
- 1 handful baby spinach, torn
- 1 onion, chopped
- 4 thyme springs, chopped
- 3 garlic cloves, minced
- 1 red bell pepper, chopped
- 1 green bell pepper, chopped
- 3 tablespoons olive oil
- 1 cup cherry tomatoes, halved
- 1 red chili pepper, chopped

Directions:

1. Heat a pan with the ghee over medium-high heat, add the eggs and some black pepper, stir, cook for 5 minutes, the add the spinach. Stir, cook for 2-3 minutes more and divide between plates.

2. Heat up another pan with the oil over medium-high heat, add the onion, stir and cook for 3 minutes. Add garlic, thyme, tomatoes, red, yellow pepper, and chili pepper, stir, cook for 5 minutes more and divide over the omelet.

3. Serve hot for breakfast.

Nutritional value/serving: calories 193, fat 16,2, fiber 3,1, carbs 10,4, protein 4,5

Paleo Soup and Stew Recipes

Coconut Cauliflower and Clam Cream

Preparation time: 10 minutes

Cooking time: 30 minutes

Servings: 6

Ingredients:

- 1 small cauliflower head, florets separated

- 2 tablespoons coconut oil, melted

- 2 cups chicken stock

- 2 carrots, chopped

- 1 yellow onion, chopped

- 2 sweet potatoes, chopped

- 17 ounces cooked fresh clams

- 1 celery rib, chopped

- 1 cup coconut milk

- A pinch of sea salt and black pepper

Directions:

1. Heat up a large saucepan with half of the oil over medium-high heat, add half of the onion, cauliflower, and stock, stir, bring to a boil and cook for 10 minutes.

2. Blend with an immersion blender, and transfer this to a bowl.

3. Heat up the same saucepan with the rest of the oil over medium heat, add the rest of the onion, celery, carrot, salt and black pepper, stir and cook for 10 minutes.

4. Add potato, 2 cups of the cauliflower cream, stir, bring to a boil and simmer for 10 minutes.

5. Add coconut milk, clams and the rest of the cauliflower cream, stir, cook for 2 minutes more, ladle into soup bowls and serve.

Nutritional value/serving: calories 260, fat 14,6, fiber 5,4, carbs 31,6, protein 3,7

Lemon Asparagus and Zucchini Cream

Preparation time: 10 minutes

Cooking time: 25 minutes

Servings: 3

Ingredients:

- 1 celery stick, chopped

- 1 zucchini, chopped

- 1 yellow onion, chopped

- 2 pounds asparagus, trimmed and roughly chopped

- 2 garlic cloves, minced

- Grated lemon peel from ½ lemon

- Black pepper to taste

- 2 cups water

- 1 tablespoon olive oil

Directions:

1. Put the asparagus, zucchini, celery, onion, lemon peel and garlic on a lined baking sheet, drizzle the oil,

season with black pepper, place in the oven at 400 degrees F and bake for 25 minutes.

2. Transfer these to a food processor, add the water and pulse well.

3. Transfer soup to a saucepan, heat up over medium heat for 1-2 minutes, ladle into bowls and serve right away.

Nutritional value/serving: calories 132, fat 5,2, fiber 8,2, carbs 18,6, protein 8,1

Lemon Cucumber Cream

Preparation time: 10 minutes

Cooking time: 0 minutes

Servings: 2

Ingredients:

- 2 cucumbers, chopped

- 1 cup coconut cream

- 1 garlic clove, minced

- 1 tablespoon olive oil

- 3 tablespoons lemon juice

- A pinch of sea salt and black pepper

Directions:

1. In your food processor, combine all the ingredients and pulse well.

2. Divide into soup bowls and serve cold.

Nutritional value/serving: calories 323, fat 29, fiber 4,2, carbs 18,1, protein 4,8

Coconut Sprouts Cream

Preparation time: 10 minutes

Cooking time: 20 minutes

Servings: 4

Ingredients:

- 2 tablespoons olive oil
- 1 yellow onion, chopped
- 2 pounds Brussels sprouts, trimmed and halved
- 4 cups chicken stock
- ¼ cup coconut cream
- A pinch of black pepper

Directions:

1. Heat up a large saucepan with the oil over medium high heat, add the onion, stir and cook for 3 minutes.
2. Add Brussels sprouts, stir and cook for 2 minutes.

3. Add stock and black pepper, stir, bring to a simmer and cook for 20 minutes.

4. Blend using an immersion blender, add coconut cream, stir well, ladle into bowls and serve right away and serve.

Nutritional value/serving: calories 153, fat 4,9, fiber 9,4, carbs 24,8, protein 9,1

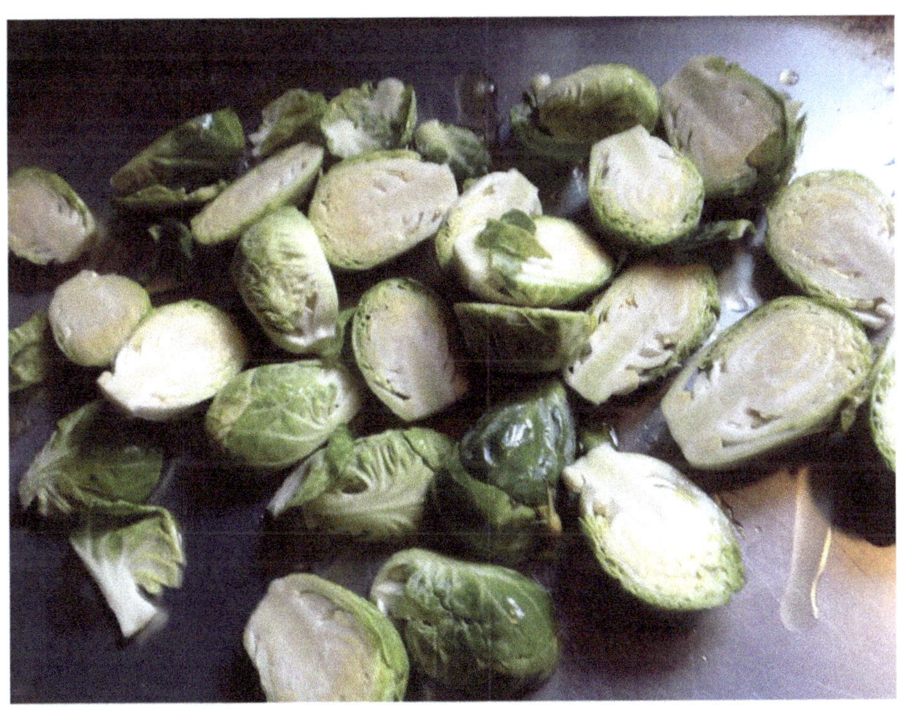

Sage Celery and Turkey Soup

Preparation time: 10 minutes

Cooking time: 30 minutes

Servings: 4

Ingredients:

- 3 and ½ cups chicken stock

- 3 tablespoons coconut oil, melted

- 1 cup coconut cream

- 3 celery stalks, chopped

- 2 carrots, chopped

- 1 sweet potato, peeled and cubed

- 2 cups turkey meat, cooked and shredded

- 1 yellow onion, chopped

- 1 tablespoon sage, chopped

- 1 teaspoon thyme, dried

- A handful parsley, chopped

- A pinch of sea salt and black pepper

Directions:

1. Heat up a large saucepan with the oil over medium heat, add celery, onions, sweet potato and carrots, stir and cook for 5 minutes.

2. Add stock, salt and pepper, stir, bring to a simmer and cook for 20 minutes.

3. Add turkey, coconut cream, sage, parsley and thyme, stir, cook for 2 minutes more, ladle into bowls and serve.

Nutritional value/serving: calories 461, fat 30,3, fiber 3,8, carbs 21,5, protein 27,6

Cashew Celery Cream

Preparation time: 10 minutes

Cooking time: 20 minutes

Servings: 2

Ingredients:

- 2 tablespoons cashews, chopped
- 17 ounces veggie stock
- A pinch of sea salt and black pepper
- 1 and ½ tablespoons olive oil
- 1 yellow onion, chopped
- 13 ounces celery, chopped

Directions:

1. Heat up a large saucepan with the oil over medium-high heat, add the onion and celery, stir and cook for 5 minutes.

2. Add stock, salt and pepper, stir, bring to a simmer and cook for 10 minutes.

3. Add cashews, stir and cook for 5 minutes more.

4. Transfer this to a blender, pulse well, divide into bowls and serve.

Nutritional value/serving: calories 181, fat 15,4, fiber 4,4, carbs 17,4, protein 3,2

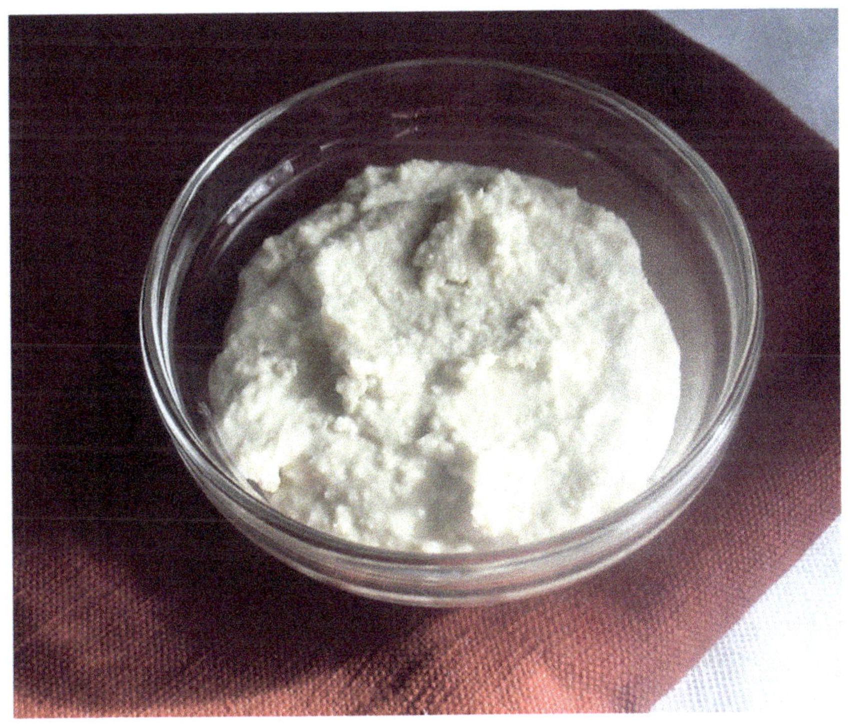

Paleo Side Dish Recipes

Lemon Broccoli

Preparation time: 10 minutes

Cooking time: 20 minutes

Servings: 4

Ingredients:

- 1 and ½ pounds broccoli

- 2 tablespoons lemon juice

- A pinch of sea salt

- 3 tablespoons avocado oil

Directions:

1. In a bowl, mix broccoli with a pinch of salt, oil and lemon juice, toss to coat well, spread on a lined

baking sheet, place in the oven at 450 degrees F and roast for 20 minutes.

2. Divide them between plates and serve.

Nutritional value/serving: calories 76, fat 1,9, fiber 5,2, carbs 12,7, protein 5,2

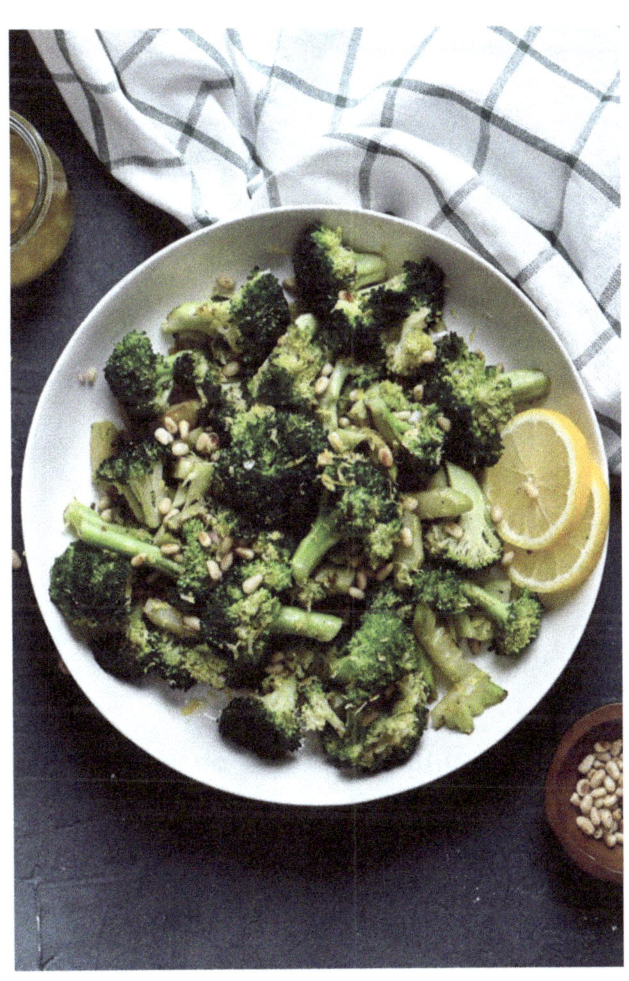

Parsley Cauliflower Mix

Preparation time: 10 minutes

Cooking time: 30 minutes

Servings: 4

Ingredients:

- 1 cauliflower head, florets separated

- ¼ cup coconut oil, melted

- ¼ cup parsley, chopped

- 2 teaspoons lemon zest, grated

- A pinch of sea salt and black pepper

- 10 garlic cloves, minced

Directions:

1. Spread cauliflower florets on a lined baking sheet, add oil and toss to coat.

2. Add a pinch of salt and black pepper, garlic, and lemon zest, toss again, place in the oven at 450 degrees F and bake for 30 minutes.

3. Sprinkle the parsley on top, toss, divide between plates and serve.

Nutritional value/serving: calories 147, fat 13,8, fiber 1,9, carbs 6,2, protein 1,9

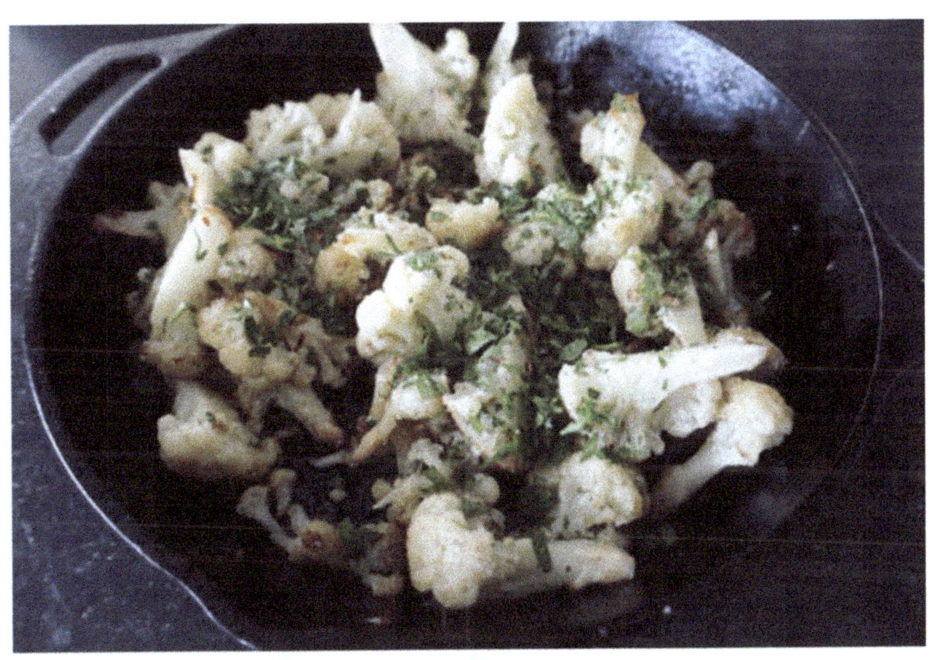

Mashed Banana Mix

Preparation time: 10 minutes

Cooking time: 30 minutes

Servings: 4

Ingredients:

- 6 ounces shallots, chopped

- 3 green bananas, peeled, halved lengthwise

- 4 garlic cloves, minced

- 1 yellow onion, chopped

- 2 tablespoons coconut oil, melted

- A pinch of sea salt

Directions:

1. Put the water in a large saucepan, bring to a boil over medium-high heat, add plantain halves, cover, cook them for 20 minutes and drain the water.

2. Heat up a pan over medium high heat, add shallots, stir and cook for 5 minutes.

3. Add garlic and onion, stir, cook for 5 minutes more, drain excess grease and transfer everything to a blender.

4. Add plantains and 2 tablespoons oil and pulse well.

5. Add a pinch of sea salt, blend again, divide between plates and serve.

Nutritional value/serving: calories 183, fat 7,2, fiber 3, carbs 30,9, protein 2,5

Kohlrani Pan

Preparation time: 10 minutes

Cooking time: 17 minutes

Servings: 3

Ingredients:

- 4 tablespoons ghee
- 3 kohlrabi, peeled and cubed
- 1 tablespoon sage, chopped
- A pinch of sea salt and black pepper

Directions:

1. Heat up a pan with the ghee over medium-high heat, add kohlrabi, a pinch of salt and black pepper, stir and cook for 15 minutes.
2. Add sage, stir again, cook for 2 minutes more, divide between plates and serve as a side dish.

Nutritional value/serving: calories 212, fat 17,3, fiber 8,4, carbs 14,4, protein 4

Sage Squash Mix

Preparation time: 10 minutes

Cooking time: 55 minutes

Servings: 4

Ingredients:

- 1 spaghetti squash, cut in halves and seeded

- 12 sage leaves, chopped

- 3 tablespoons ghee, melted

- A pinch of sea salt

- Black pepper to taste

Directions:

1. Place spaghetti squash on a lined baking sheet, place in the oven at 375 degrees F, bake for 40 minutes, and scoop strings of flesh into a bowl.

2. Heat up a pan with the ghee over medium heat, add sage, cook for 5 minutes and transfer them to paper towels.

3. Heat up the pan again over medium heat, add spaghetti squash, salt and black pepper to the taste, stir and cook for 3 minutes.

4. Add the sage, stir, divide between plates and serve as a side.

Nutritional value/serving: calories 108, fat 10,3, fiber 2, carbs 4,8, protein 0,7

Thyme Baked Squash

Preparation time: 10 minutes

Cooking time: 35 minutes

Servings: 6

Ingredients:

- 2 tablespoons coconut oil, melted
- 2 pounds butternut squash, peeled, seeded and cubed
- 2 teaspoons thyme, chopped
- A pinch of black pepper

Directions

1. In a bowl, mix squash cubes with oil, thyme, and pepper and toss to combine.
2. Spread them on a lined baking sheet, place in the oven at 425 degrees F and bake for 35 minutes.
3. Divide between plates and serve as a side dish.

Nutritional value/serving: calories 108, fat 4,7, fiber 3,1, carbs 17,9, protein 1,5

Paleo Meat Recipes

Herbed Lamb Mix

Preparation time: 10 minutes

Cooking time: 20 minutes

Servings: 4

Ingredients:

- 2 garlic cloves, minced
- 1 tablespoon lemon zest
- 1 tablespoon oregano, chopped
- 8 lamb chops
- 2/3 cup olive oil
- 1/3 cup basil, chopped
- 2 tablespoons balsamic vinegar
- A pinch of sea salt
- Black pepper to taste

- 3 tablespoons Dijon mustard

Directions:

1. In a bowl, mix oil with oregano, garlic and lemon zest and whisk well.

2. Brush lamb chops with this mix, season them with salt and black pepper to taste, place them on preheated grill over medium-high heat and cook for 5 minutes on each side.

3. In a bowl, mix mustard with a pinch of salt, basil, vinegar and black pepper and whisk well.

4. Divide lamb chops on plates, drizzle mint sauce over them and serve.

Nutritional value/serving: calories 1521, fat 82,2, fiber 1, carbs 2,3, protein 184,5

Cumin Lamb

Preparation time: 10 minutes

Cooking time: 2 hours and 30 minutes

Servings: 4

Ingredients:

- 15 garlic cloves, peeled

- 2 teaspoons onion powder

- 6 lamb shanks

- 2 teaspoons cumin powder

- 1 cup water

- 3 teaspoons oregano, dried

- ½ cup olive oil

- A pinch of sea salt and black pepper

- ½ cup lemon juice

Directions:

1. In a roasting pan, combine all the ingredients, toss well and roast in the oven at 350 degrees F for 2

hours and 30 minutes.

2. Divide everything between plates and serve.

Nutritional value/serving: calories 647, fat 41,4, fiber 1, carbs 6,5, protein 61,1

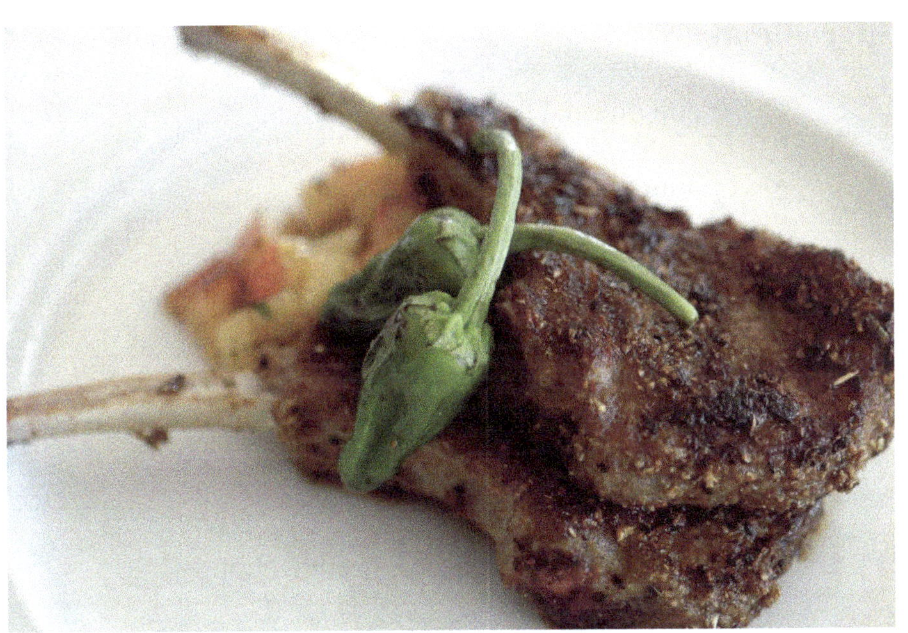

Turkey with Tomatoes

Preparation time: 10 minutes

Cooking time: 1 hour and 10 minutes

Servings: 6

Ingredients:

- ¼ cup onion, chopped
- 1 pound turkey meat, ground
- 1 sweet potato, cut with a spiralizer
- 1 eggplant, chopped
- 1 tablespoon garlic, minced
- 8 ounces tomato paste
- 12 ounces fresh tomatoes, peeled, chopped
- A pinch of sea salt and black pepper
- ¼ teaspoon chili powder
- ¼ teaspoon cumin, ground
- Cooking spray
- ½ teaspoon tarragon flakes

For the sauce:

- 1 tablespoon coconut flour
- 1 tablespoon almond flour
- 1 cup almond milk
- 1 and ½ tablespoons olive oil

Directions:

1. Heat up a pan over medium heat, add onion, turkey and garlic, stir and brown for a few minutes.

2. Add tomatoes, tomato paste and sweet potatoes, stir and cook for a few minutes more.

3. In a bowl, mix eggplant pieces with a pinch of sea salt, black pepper, chili powder, cumin and tarragon flakes and stir well.

4. Spread eggplant into a baking dish after greased with cooking spray, top with the turkey mix, place in the oven at 350 degrees F and bake for 15 minutes.

5. Heat up a pan with the oil over medium heat, add coconut and almond flour and stir for 1 minute.

6. Add almond milk and cook for 10 minutes stirring often.

7. Top the turkey casserole with this sauce, place in the oven again and bake for 40 minutes more.

8. Slice and serve hot.

Nutritional value/serving: calories 307, fat 13,9, fiber 6,6, carbs 21, protein 26,5

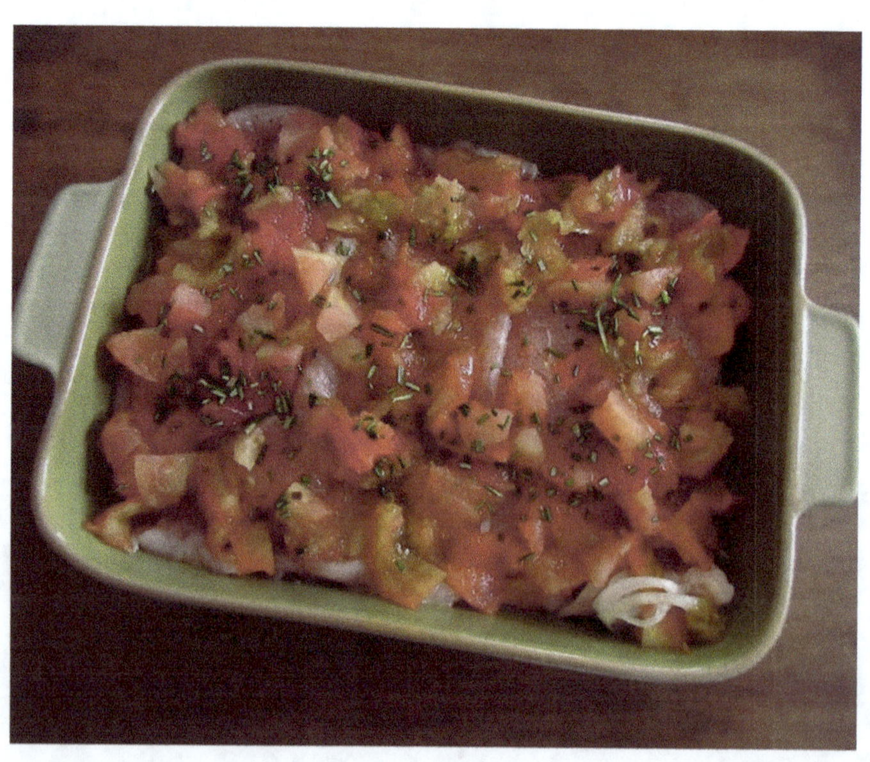

Beef Cakes

Preparation time: 10 minutes

Cooking time: 25 minutes

Servings: 4

Ingredients:

- 2 sweet potatoes, boiled and grated
- 1 pound beef, ground
- 1 cup red onion, chopped
- 2 Serrano peppers, chopped
- 1-inch ginger piece, grated
- A handful cilantro, chopped
- 4 garlic cloves, minced
- ½ teaspoon meat masala
- A pinch of cayenne pepper
- ¼ teaspoon turmeric powder
- Black pepper to taste
- 1 egg, whisked

- 4 tablespoons almond meal

- 1 cup water

- 5 tablespoons ghee, melted

Directions:

1. Heat up a pan over medium high heat, add beef, masala, turmeric, black pepper and cayenne pepper, stir and brown for 5 minutes.

2. Add the water, stir, cook for 10 minutes more and take off heat.

3. Heat up another pan with 2 tablespoons ghee over medium heat, add Serrano peppers and onion, stir and cook for 2 minutes.

4. Add garlic and ginger, stir and cook for 1 minute more.

5. Add cilantro and the meat mixture, stir well and take off heat.

6. Add grated sweet potatoes, stir well, cool everything down and shape patties from this mix.

7. Put the egg in a bowl and almond meal in another.

8. Dredge the patties in egg and then in almond meal.

9. Heat up a pan with the rest of the ghee over medium heat, add beef patties, cook them for 4 minutes on each side and divide between plates.

10. Serve them with a side salad.

Nutritional value/serving: calories 512, fat 27,3, fiber 5, carbs 27,2, protein 39,1

Cilantro Beef Mix

Preparation time: 10 minutes

Cooking time: 35 minutes

Servings: 4

Ingredients:

- 1 pound beef, ground
- 1 teaspoon cumin seeds, toasted
- 1 pound sweet potatoes, cubed
- 3 tablespoons ghee
- 2 onions, chopped
- 1 small ginger pieces, grated
- 1 Serrano pepper, chopped
- 2 teaspoons coriander powder
- 2 teaspoons garam masala
- Black pepper to the taste
- 1 cup steamed broccoli
- A handful cilantro, chopped

Directions:

1. Heat up a pan with 2 tablespoons ghee over medium heat, add sweet potato cubes, stir, cook them for 20 minutes and transfer them to a bowl.

2. Heat up the same pan over medium heat, add cumin, Serrano pepper and onion, stir and cook for 4 minutes.

3. Add beef, ginger, coriander, garam masala, cayenne and black pepper, stir and cook for 5 minutes more.

4. Add broccoli and sweet potatoes, stir, cook for 5 minutes more, divide between plates and serve with cilantro on top.

Nutritional value/serving: calories 465, fat 17,1, fiber 6,8, carbs 39,4, protein 37,8

Beef Stir Fry

Preparation time: 10 minutes

Cooking time: 15 minutes

Servings: 4

Ingredients:

- 1 yellow onion, chopped
- 1 pound beef, ground
- 1 napa cabbage head, shredded
- 1 carrot, grated
- A pinch of sea salt
- Black pepper to taste
- 2 tablespoons coconut oil, melted

Directions:

1. Heat up a pan with the oil over medium-high heat, add the onion and beef, stir and brown them for 5 minutes.

2. Add carrots, cabbage, a pinch of salt and black pepper to taste, stir and cook for 10 minutes more.

3. Divide between plates and serve.

Nutritional value/serving: calories 314, fat 14,3, fiber 3,1, carbs 8,7, protein 38

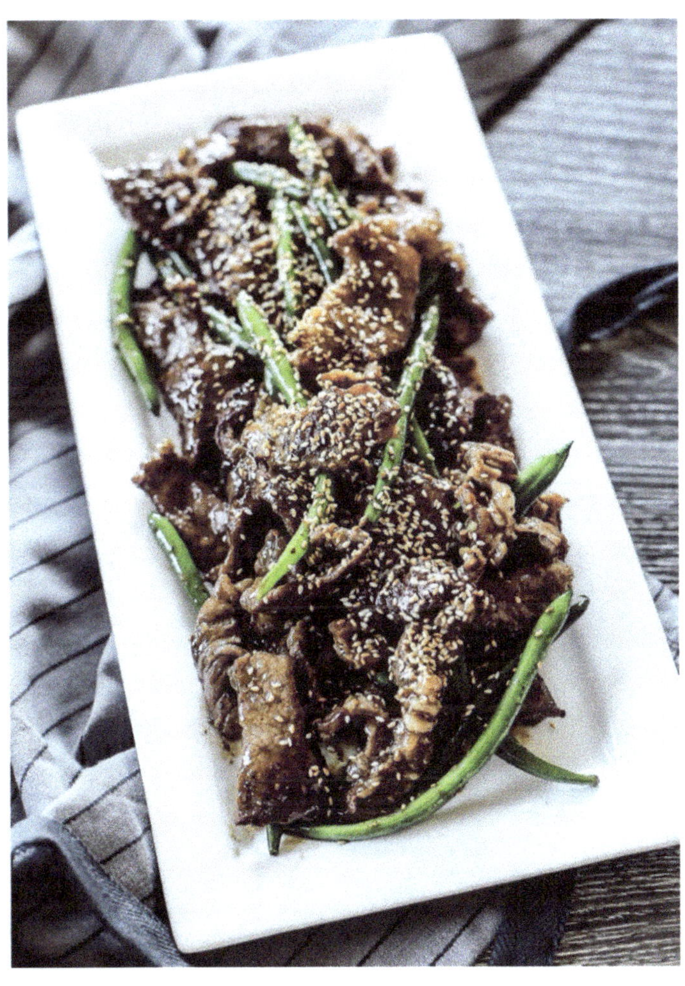